ADHD
SUPERPOWER
II

*Making Use of the
Power of ADHD*

Introduction.............................8

Chapter 1: What is ADHD?..........12
- ADD and ADHD – What's the
Difference?...............................14
- What are the Symptoms of ADHD?....16
- Fire, Ready, Aim –
- A Mind Out of Order........................20

**Chapter 2: Is it Really a Curse or is
it a Gift?.....................................23**
- Changing Perceptions About ADHD. .24
- ADHD is Not the Problem..................29
- Why It Can be a Gift..........................30

**Chapter 3: Finding the Power
Within...33**
- Creating the Right Profile to Enhance
Your Gift...............................33
- Balancing Work and Family...............37
- Find Activities That You Both Can Be
Excited About.....................................42
- Strategies to Help You Go from Off
Beat to On Point.................................42
- For Disorganization:........................43
- To Control Impulsive Tendencies......44
- To Manage Stress............................45
- Finding Your Power in Nature..........46
- Channel That Surplus Energy...........48

Chapter 4: Thinking Differently..51
- Self-Soothing Techniques...................53

- Dare to Use Your Emotions...............55
- Principles to Live By........................57

Chapter 5: Managing Your Time With ADHD.................................59
- Time Management in Everyday Situations.......................................59
- Set Time Management Goals.............61

Chapter 6: Taking it to the Next Level...64
- Allow for Distractions......................65
- Give the Business a Direction...........66
- You Can Wear Several Hats, but Don't 66
- Use Your Visual Cues......................67
- What Kind of Business to Start?.......67

The information in the following pages is broadly considered to be a truthful and accurate account of facts and as such any inattention, use or misuse of the information in question by the reader will render any resulting actions solely under their purview. There are no scenarios in which the publisher or the original author of this work can be in any fashion deemed liable for any hardship or damages that may befall them after undertaking information described herein.

Additionally, the information in the following pages is intended only for informational purposes and should thus be thought of as universal. As befitting its nature, it is presented without assurance regarding its prolonged validity or interim quality. Trademarks that are mentioned are done without written consent and can in no way be considered an endorsement from the trademark holder.

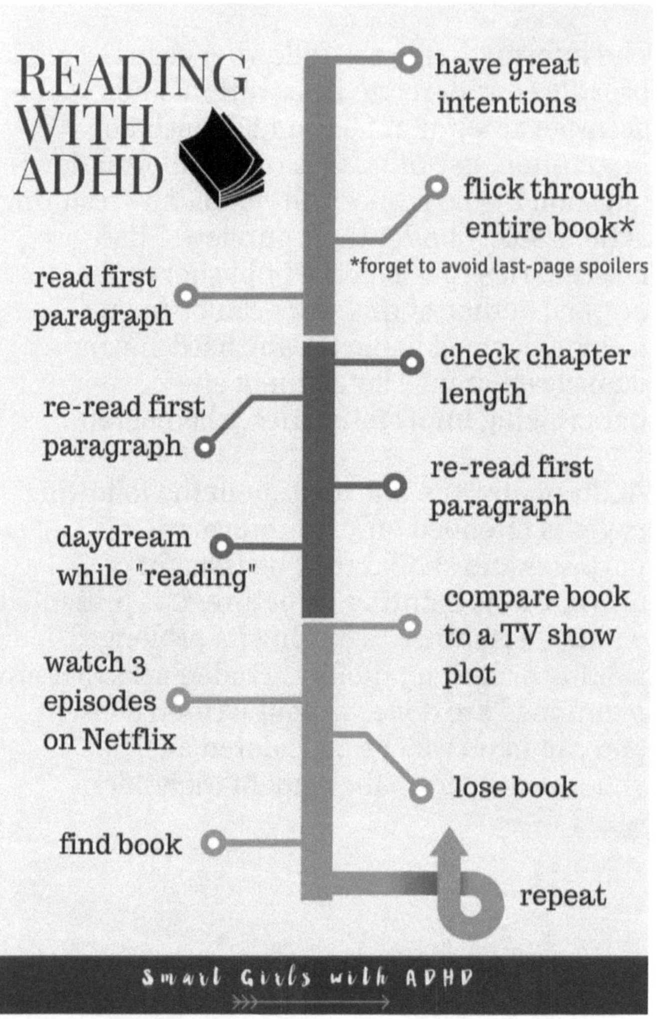

READING WITH ADHD
have great intentions
flick through entire book*
*forget to avoid last-page spoilers
read first paragraph
check chapter length
re-read first paragraph
re-read first paragraph
daydream while "reading"
compare book to a TV show plot
watch 3 episodes on Netflix
lose book
find book
repeat
Smart Girls with ADHD

Introduction

Congratulations on buying this book and thank you for doing so.

The cry of epidemic has been sweeping the nation for at least a decade if not more. The condition that has touched on nearly every household in the nation is not some infectious disease that slowly grows inside the body to the point that little else can be survive its relentless assault. It's not some bacteria that slowly eats away at one's vital systems, and it's not some failure of the heart condition that stops the body's circulation in its tracks.

No, the disease is not that recognizable and yet people everywhere are calling it an epidemic of mass proportions. It is a "disease" of the mind, one that has been classified as a mental health disorder that has parents running to the pharmacies to get their hyperactive children under control. It has adults lying on the psychiatrist's couch in hopes of triggering some thought or seed buried deep in their mind that will bring them a sense of calm.

Being diagnosed with ADHD has always been met with increasing alarm over the years. The idea that something is wrong with the mind can be a frightening thing even for an adult. On the one hand, it gives a sense of relief when you realize that you are not just lazy, irresponsible, or aloof but there is actually a scientific explanation for your behavior.

But now, as we learn more and more about ADHD, it is becoming clearer than ever that sometimes thinking differently is just that, someone who actually does think differently. Classifying it as a disorder could turn out to be an epic injustice perpetrated on millions of people every year. Because someone thinks "differently" doesn't necessarily mean there is something wrong with them, it simply means that their thoughts may not completely jive with the mainstream population.

This type of debate as to whether ADHD should continue to be classified as a "disorder" or not will probably rage on for many more years. However, in the interim, there have been many strides that have been helpful in teaching those who are afflicted with ADHD how to cope with the way their minds work.

Today, there is an entire subset of the world's population that are discovering that the names they have been labeled with are not necessarily a curse as many were led to believe but are in fact a real blessing. Their minds, unique as they are, have been equipped with an entirely different way of processing information. To that end, they don't all need to have drugs to help them manage their lives. They've discovered the drugs have been used primarily so they could fit into the old traditional modes of society, but once they have been removed, they are finding their unique thought processes can literally give them a decided advantage, which is the focus of this book you are reading now.

In the following chapters you'll learn just how you can turn a negative diagnosis of ADHD into something positive.

You will learn:

- What ADHD is
- How to use your mental capabilities to your advantage
- How to create an environment that is conducive to your growth
- Helpful strategies that will help you to tap into your natural thinking process
- How to keep your emotions in balance when you live against the grain
- How to manage time when you're constantly distracted
- How to choose the right work environment best suited for you
- And what to do if you should decide to strike out on your own

This book is not about identifying another disability and giving you tools to live with it. Instead, it is about embracing the differences and teaching you how to live your life in a positive and affirmative way. If that is a goal

that you want for those with ADHD, then it's
time for us to get started.

There are plenty of books on this subject on the
market, thanks again for choosing this one!
Every effort was made to ensure it is full of as
much useful information as possible, please
enjoy!

<u>Chapter 1</u>: What is ADHD?

Everyone experiences a break in our concentration from time to time. Our state of consciousness can vary from those early morning waking up periods all the way up to a hyper focus at other times. This is perfectly normal and adjustments to these variations are relatively easy for most people.

Many with ADHD are able to shift between these varying states of attentiveness quickly and easily. It doesn't take a lot of structure or planning; their brains just shift gears in much the same way an automatic car's transmission does. The adjustment is barely noticeable. They can shift from a hyper focused state of mind and back to normal then shift down to a near vegetative state and back with no problem at all.

However, for a very small percentage of people, this ability to shift comes far too easily. They find it difficult to sit and tune into an object or zero in on a task for an extended period of time. At the other end of the spectrum, they could also slip into that almost catatonic state and end up straddled with an almost paralyzing inability to function or move even the slightest. Once they fall into either of these mental states it is a fight to snap back to the normalcy that the average person can do so easily. When they do, they may find it extremely difficult to stay focused on anything for any length of time. Sometimes, their mind will wander aimlessly after only a few seconds on task and other times it could be so in tuned that it is difficult to pull them off point. It is for these people that this book is written. Those people who can't control their mental wanderings and have difficulty pulling themselves back from the brink of oblivion from one moment to the next.

As a child, they were diagnosed as having a mental disorder called ADD or ADHD. Many seem to grow out of it when they become adults, but new theories seem to show that rather than "grow out of it" they instead learn how to use it. As a child, they were probably labeled as unmotivated by teachers and lazy by well-meaning parents. This inability to focus was often coupled with uncontrollable bursts of energy that propelled them to move at some of the most inopportune times. As children, there was the frustration of teachers and administrators alike. They found it difficult to do the boring and mundane tasks often asked of many students. Once they mastered a skill, their sense of accomplishment was over and they were all ready to learn something else, something new and different.

As adults, this condition presents itself in different ways. They may find themselves unable to take on a task and stick to it for hours or days at a time. They may have good days where everything they do is right and days when everything they do is wrong. At times, it may not be an issue of what is right or wrong but the order of the way they do things or their inability to complete tasks based on the standards of the corporate hierarchy. As a result of their inability to conform, many lose their jobs and find themselves bouncing from one job to the next feeling more and more disconnected with each passing failure. This is what life is like as an adult with ADHD.

ADD and ADHD – What's the Difference?

ADHD has been one of the most commonly diagnosed childhood disorders for years. The terms ADD and ADHD are often used interchangeably in many situations and while in the past, we thought we understood the condition, with additional research, more information has helped all of us to get a much clearer grasp of both terms.

In the past, ADD meant Attention Deficit Disorder, but that reference is now considered outdated. It was a designation for someone who had difficulty focusing and staying on task but was not hyperactive; they lacked the impulsiveness of the condition. In this understanding, those with ADD would simply struggle to keep their minds focused on the task at hand and would have no other symptoms relating to the disorder.

Today, after many years of careful research, our understanding of the condition is so much better. The term ADD, while still being used, is no longer a primary designation of the condition. Instead, the term ADHD (Attention Deficit Hyperactivity Disorder) is used for all cases. There are now three different types of ADHD that you may be diagnosed with.

What Does the Diagnostic and Statistical Manual of Mental Health Disorders Say?

When mental health professionals diagnose someone with ADHD, they usually refer to a very specific set of symptoms detailed in *The Diagnostic and Statistical Manual of Mental Disorders*. This book, published by the American Psychiatric Association, provides a detailed list of criteria they can use to identify a wide range of mental disorders.

One of the most significant changes in the DSM over the years is that ADHD is no longer considered a childhood disorder. Instead, as the child matures, the condition takes on different forms, symptoms change, and responses can vary depending on the age.

The DSM describes it s a "neurodevelopmental disorder" evidenced by a pattern of inattention

accompanied by hyperactivity in some cases.
The degree to which someone may struggle
with this order can cause a negative impact to
their daily lives in work, relationships, and
social situations.

The good news about this new designation is
that now the field is wide open for many other
people to get the attention and treatment they
deserve to help them to manage the condition.
In the past, since its focus was entirely
concentrated on children; many teens and
adults that showed symptoms of ADHD were
completely disregarded or problem cases and
often fell through the cracks. Now, with studies
expanded to incorporate these older
individuals, we have an even clearer
understanding of how ADHD works and have a
more effective way of managing it.

What are the Symptoms of ADHD?

There are three different types of ADHD we
should all be aware of.

- **Inattentive:**

This is a person who demonstrates symptoms of
inattention or inability to focus for what could
be considered a normal period of time on a
given task. They are easily distracted but they

do not show signs of impulsiveness or hyperactivity.

Common symptoms of someone with Inattentive ADHD can include:

1. Easily distracted
2. Often forgets even regular daily tasks
3. Inability to concentrate on work or other activities
4. Makes frequent mistakes
5. Mentally fades out even when spoken to directly
6. Often fails to follow instructions
7. Often has incomplete tasks
8. Loses focus/daydreaming
9. Is disorganized
10. Tendency to avoid tasks that require long periods of mental effort
11. Frequently loses things

- **Hyperactive/Impulsive:**

This is a person that shows symptoms of
hyperactivity and impulsiveness but no
signs of inattentiveness.

Common symptoms of someone with
Hyperactivity/Impulsive ADHD:

1. Always needing to move
2. Excessive talking
3. Impatient – struggles to wait for things
4. Unable to sit still – tapping hands or feet – fidgety
5. Constantly moving even in inappropriate situations
6. Difficulty relaxing even in leisure activities
7. Speaks over other people, interrupts conversations even before the other person finishes speaking
8. Constantly intruding on others
9. May struggle to keep their emotions in check

- **Combined**

Combined ADHD is a combination of
both inattentiveness along with the
hyperactivity and impulsiveness.

There are quite a few more symptoms to look for to demonstrate ADHD but these are enough to help you determine if you should see a professional in order to find out if you or someone close to you has ADHD.

Of course, all people have these conditions at one time or another but a true person with ADHD will consistently demonstrate these symptoms in their lives. Someone who misplaces their keys once in a blue moon is not likely to have ADHD but if they lose their keys with regularity it could be evidence of the condition.

According to the DSM-5 if six or more of these symptoms are present in a child, they could be diagnosed with ADHD. In those over the age of 17, they should have at least five of these symptoms.

Fire, Ready, Aim – A Mind Out of Order

Understanding the definition of ADHD doesn't necessarily help you to fully grasp its impact. Living with ADHD can be a totally different experience. Yes, it helps to put a label on the problem, explain why you don't fit in with so many perfectly normal situations but knowledge doesn't alleviate the challenges that are faced on a daily basis.

Imagine a young student in school assigned to read a full chapter of a history textbook overnight, or the adult businessman who must read a new business proposal before the next corporate meeting. They both love to read, they both want to do it, but the size of the task is overwhelming for someone with ADHD.

The true problem they face is not even the size of the task, it is how their brain is working. Some have described it as a sort of "brain fog" that makes it difficult to see through to what really needs to be done. It can be like a motor running inside their heads that doesn't want to shut off, constantly changing gears, often out of order. The idea of sitting through a single task for hours at a time can literally be frightening for someone with ADHD. It is difficult to control the urge to change gears, move, or redirect their focus.

When speaking to others, without warning
their brains will shift gears and their minds will
no longer hear what's being said. Sitting for 45
minutes to an hour in a meeting can be a real
struggle. They may be eager to volunteer for a
project, but their mind is on the end result.
Later when it is time to put a plan into action,
they realize how much of a commitment they
have agreed to. The stages of work for them are
to think about the end as if it were already
completed, then go back and prepare, and
finally actually doing the work.

In many cases, this disorganized brain process
can be treated with medication, but there are
thousands, if not millions of people the world
over, who have never been officially diagnosed
who have developed strategies to help them
navigate the murky regions of their brain. They
still struggle to see through the fog but at least
now they have developed a plan that will help
them to cope with activities that most people
would consider perfectly normal.

Whether you decide to treat your out of order
brain with medication or manage your
symptoms with something else, the primary
focus here is to have a plan. Those that don't
develop some method of bringing their thought
process back in line with the world around
them will end up searching for solutions in
other areas of their lives. Many drop out of
school from frustration and discouragement,

some will turn to illegal drugs or other
practices to help them cope, which could
compound the problem rather than helping it.

Aside from medications to calm the confused
spirit, people have also turned to other forms of
therapy to help them including cognitive
behavioral therapy or CBT. Whatever you
decide to do, the key point here is to develop a
positive plan of action that will allow your
thought process to settle down, at least for a
little while, so that you will be able to function
in a world that doesn't always recognize what's
going on inside your head.

Chapter 2: Is it Really a Curse or is it a Gift?

Interestingly enough, the more we learn about ADHD the more people are beginning to believe that it is not a true disorder. The different thought process does not always translate into something wrong.

We can better understand this by looking at the way the world is set up. Much like the IQ test is designed primarily for those with certain skills, it is not a true measure of intelligence in all areas of society. Yes, the IQ test will measure your ability to solve puzzles, math problems, and read extensive passages in textbooks, but that intelligence means nothing if you're riding up a crocodile invested river in the Amazon forest. Just like intelligence is relative to your environment, the same can be said of those with ADHD. There are definitely unique environments where those with ADHD can thrive as opposed to others.

The challenge is to find that spot and that area where the mental faculties and skills of the ADHD person are in fact a gift rather than a curse.

Changing Perceptions About ADHD

Rather than viewing ADHD as a curse, perceptions need to be changed. When it is thought of as a curse, a negative vibe runs through the community. However, there is no question that those with ADHD have a unique way of viewing the world around them. Their constant mental "jumping" from one thought to the next can help them to be more alert to certain conditions, more in tuned to warning signs, can make them much more efficient in certain areas of work.

The sad truth however, is that within certain environments, it can be very difficult to know what the public perception of the condition truly is. It is difficult to control what other people may say about you, let alone what they may think but over time, the negative perception of ADHD will eventually give way to more positive thinking.

In many cases, those with ADHD are often misunderstood and therefore cast aside as a problem that needs to be ignored or at the very least delegated to a lower role. This creates a huge challenge for the adult with ADHD.

Some of the common misconceptions that many have are that those with ADHD can be problematic and difficult to communicate with.

You can imagine what kind of problems that type of preconceived notion can have on an adult with the ADHD experience in the workplace. People will view them in a negative light regardless of how well they perform their jobs.

This image can follow them throughout their lives causing them a battery of problems along the way. Many have lost jobs, broken relationships, and a host of other issues they must face with that are completely beyond the scope of their control.

We see signs of this in certain situations. For example, a person with ADHD may have a mind drift right at a crucial point in a business meeting, which could cost them dearly later on. They may have missed out on valuable information so even if they were to resume their attention minutes later, the points they may have missed could create major complications. To the other people involved, it could be viewed as an inability to understand, perceived as a lack of interest or dedication to the job, or any number of negative reactions. The sad truth is that very few will attribute it to their ADHD and will thus label them according to their own perceptions. In either situation, it is not an easy situation to cope with for either party. The challenge that must be faced here is not just teaching the person with ADHD how to cope with their condition but helping those without ADHD to change their own perceptions so that both will have a positive experience in their interactions.

These kinds of situations can repeat themselves in different scenarios over and over again throughout the course of one's life. The trick in changing perceptions about them lies in developing specific strategies that will help them to cope with these "misses" by doing some of the following. Keep in mind that we'll discuss some of these strategies in more detail in later chapters of the book, but these listed below are perfect for helping to get started in changing the world's perceptions about how to interact with those with ADHD.

- Avoid punishing yourself for failure to perform when your ADHD is the problem. This will only compound the problem and inset feelings of guilt and shame into your process.
- Don't accept the labels that many people will give you. Often those with ADHD will have a self protecting mechanism that will be triggered when problems arise. They may be called manipulative, undependable, or even liars in certain situations. Don't give in to those labels and don't accept them as part of your true nature.
- Keep in mind that you're dealing with a neurological issue, the actions are not intentional.

- Rather than just making verbal promises, try to show enthusiasm for your work and your goal for doing the right thing whenever it is in your power to do so.
- Whenever it is appropriate, make sure that those around you know that you have ADHD and you may lose your focus or become confused in certain situations. Because of all of the previous misconceptions, you won't want to tell everyone, but you can be the judge of situations when you feel it could serve to your benefit to let your coworkers or employers know of your ADHD and what they can do to make the process run smoother for everyone.
- Whenever possible, educate others about ADHD and what's in or out of your control.
- Encourage written records of conversations and interactions as a means of backing up your actions. Make sure this is done in a collaborative way rather than taking the adversarial approach.
- Be sensitive to other's limitations and show empathy. You may be dealing with ADHD, but they may be dealing with other issues as well. A good show of fellow feeling can go a long way in smoothing things out in the environment.

If you don't have ADHD but you have to
interact with someone who does on a
regular basis, here are a few suggestions
that could help you to change perceptions
as well.

- Exercise patience and a calm spirit
  and avoid passing your frustrations
  on to them.
- Avoid the temptation to punish them
  for their failings. It will only create
  more resistance, which will create
  more problems in the future.
- Show empathy and understanding
  whenever possible.
- Recognize their courage for
  continuing to repeatedly try in spite
  of the situation.
- Be willing to create written records
  of conversations and interactions.
- Ask for them to repeat and clarify
  information when they give it.
- Be sincere and give praise whenever
  deserved.
- Be willing to learn more about
  ADHD and how best to communicate
  with them.
- Keep in mind that ADHD is not a
  choice but your decision to be
  flexible is. Being tolerant and
  understanding can make a huge
  difference in how smoothly any given
  situation will go.

ADHD is Not the Problem

As we learn more about ADHD many are beginning to realize that it may not actually be a disorder at all. The mind of the ADHD person simply processes information and thinks completely differently than other minds that are considered normal.

According to several studies, ADHD makes up the second most frequent long-term diagnosis in America followed only by asthma. This condition alone generates more than $9 billion of pharmaceutical sales every year. All of this is in light of the fact that it has never been declared an authentic "illness" in the clinical term of the word.

The reality is that ADHD is not the problem, being different is the problem. In fact, many researchers are now struggling to come to terms with even calling it an abnormality. Instead, they see a diagnosis of ADHD as a means of labeling unwanted or undesirable behavior rather than an actual condition that must be treated.

If this theory is true, the fact that a person with ADHD actually thinks differently means that there is no true problem to deal with. Instead, the focus should be on how different parties can work to build communication and work together in a wide range of environments. Diagnosing ADHD as a "disorder" would then

be tantamount to saying that one form of
normal is more valid or important than
another. The reality is simple, there is room for
all different types of thinking ability so if you're
someone with ADHD, labeling is not going to
help you as much as learning which
environments, work situations, and strategies
will help you to blend well with others in your
immediate society.

Why It Can be a Gift

It may seem strange to call ADHD a real gift
but once you learn how to channel that energy,
to take advantage of the many thoughts
running through your mind and learn how to
tap into the natural resourcefulness it creates,
you'll have a wonderful assemblage of skills
and creativity that can be applied in a wide
range of situations.

While the "normal" thinker may have the
ability to stay on one task for hours on end, the
versatility and the ability of the ADHD mind to
switch midstreams may actually prove more
beneficial in many environments.

It is true that adults with ADHD tend to have
more divorces, lose jobs more often, and even
can drift into cases of drug and alcohol abuse,
they also have a whole new set of skills that
when put to the right use, many will envy.

Those with ADHD can be very entertaining, uninhibited, and creative, definitely have strong suits in many different ways.

In the right situations, they can be a spark of life in an otherwise painfully boring business meeting. They can provide a burst of energy in an otherwise mundane affair. They are resilient, inventive, intuitive, and when on task, during those moments when their minds are in tune with what's before them can demonstrate amazing powers of hyper focus that would be difficult for most others to compete with.

All of these qualities can be a curse, but they can also be a gift. Those who are most successful know how to take these innate skills and turn them into emotional intelligence that can go so much further than an IQ.

To make that happen though, there are some pretty basic skills that they must master. They need to figure out how to follow through on tasks when their minds are disoriented, they need to hone their organizational skills, and they need to bring a bit more discipline and training into their lives.

We all have impulses that we want to follow; the ADHD person needs to learn how to not give into them at every turn. If they can master the skill of delayed gratification and follow through, many the perceived drawbacks of ADHD can suddenly be channeled in a new direction creating a wealth of skills and gifts that can take them very far in their everyday interactions of life.

The secret therein lies in how you control your environment. Finding the right place to expend your skills is key to using these gifts. If you're hyper and you have a job staring at a computer screen for hours on end, chances are your extra energy is not going to be a gift. However, if you find a career that allows you to jump up, move around, multi-task with a flexible work when you can schedule, you're going to love having ADHD. In fact, you just might want to brag about it.

The reality is that the world is now changing in favor of those with ADHD. Our time in this age of technology allows and actually expects us to multi-task in just about every aspect of our lives. Jobs are now flexible enough that you can work from home, set your own schedule, and even do several jobs at one time. The skills needed for these new careers of the modern age are the very same ones that are instinctive for someone with ADHD. Even the impetuousness that got you into trouble as a child can turn into a curiosity to experience all the new innovations introduced in the world today. Properly channeled, they could put you on the leading edge of industry in society.

Chapter 3: Finding the Power Within

To take your unique talents of ADHD and use them to your advantage there are a few things you will need to do first. You need to claim the power to shape your own life. Gone are the days when you had to cow-tow to an employer's every whim. In this modern age, your work and life environment can be exactly what you want it to be as long as you take the initiative to claim that power for yourself.

This requires a certain amount of courage. You may find that you have to go against the grain of society, but if you do, you can create a life that is perfectly suited to your impulsiveness and constant bursts of energy. This means you become the master of your universe rather than allowing the universe to control you. You must take the initiative to create your own world that is perfectly suited to your unique set of strengths and weaknesses.

Creating the Right Profile to Enhance Your Gift

If you were diagnosed with ADHD a long time ago, you may not even realize the unlimited number of options you have at your disposal. The world has changed a great deal in the past twenty years. You no longer have to be glued to a desk in a classroom for 6 hours a day nor do you have to be glued to an office cubicle for 8 hours a day any longer. With the increasing popularity of homeschooling and work at home programs, you can choose the lifestyle you want in pretty much the same way you would order a meal at a restaurant.

This is good news for anyone with ADHD because now they can pick and choose the environment they want to spend their days in. They are free to find work that will allow them to make the most of their unique skills and talents. Rather than trying to find a situation that will tolerate your ADHD, you can create a situation that will make the most of it.

This may not be so easy to do, though. The idea of "fitting in" to society is so deeply engrained into each of us that it can be a little scary to step outside of the accepted norms and demand your own piece of the world. However, once you have broken free from those preconceived ideas, you will find it quite refreshing to live life the way you were meant to.

Taking the first step in this regard will require you to do some soul searching. You need to determine what things you are passionate about and create a plan that will help you bring more of them into your routine. You can start by making a list of things you really enjoy doing and what types of situations you find yourself comfortable in. This may require you to do a little research to find out possible opportunities that are available now, but if it is something that you are passionate about, it won't seem like an unnecessary chore.

Keep in mind that you are pushing out the old way of doing things and starting in on the new. Unlike in school where in order to succeed, you needed to be a little expert in everything. You needed to be able to master algebra, geometry, geography, and history in order to move on to the next level.

Today though, you can bypass most things you're not comfortable doing. You can choose a profession where your strong suits are enhanced, and the other skills are not as important. You don't need to be a master of everything under the sun. Once you discover your true strengths and passions, creating that profile environment you want will be easy and once you start the ball to rolling, you'll just fall right into step with your new life.

Realize that now, with so many options at your disposal, your profile can truly allow you to thrive. Those with ADHD generally do best with jobs that demand a lot of mobility which could range from something as basic as automobile mechanics to machine operators, police officers, firefighters, nursery workers, construction workers, wait staff, landscaping, dancers, musicians, actors, journalists, tree fallers, athletes, and you get the idea.

Think about these careers and what they require. They don't need you to be able to recite all the states in America in alphabetical order nor do they demand that you memorize long passages of prose and recite it back to your employer. Instead, they require energy, dedication, passion, and the ability solve problems when they arise; all skills naturally inherent in people with ADHD.

This means a change in how you think about yourself. For years, you've probably been told something is wrong with you, now you have to start thinking in terms of "what is right with me?" The most successful ADHD worker is the one who is willing to create the life that enhances their strong suits rather than trying to fit themselves into an environment full of people that don't understand them and situations that won't allow them to make the most of their talents.

Look for situations that will provide you with constant stimulation, a frequent change of pace, and the ability to create and use your talents. These will naturally meet your needs and make your feel more relaxed. By doing this, you create a profile environment that will take you to a whole new way of living your life.

Balancing Work and Family

In creating your new environment, you also need to find a happy balance between your new work life and your family life. Chances are as you embark on this new "build my own profile" project your life will become more chaotic. This is not a challenge that only those with ADHD struggle with. In most cases, people in general will be in a constant battle for balancing both very important aspects of their lives.

However, it is a much more difficult problem for those with ADHD. Because many struggle with self-regulation, it can be very difficult to balance your life between the two. While difficult though, it is not impossible. This will become even more difficult if you decide to take on a work at home job.

If you're single and living alone, it may not be as complicated a process as someone with a spouse and children running afoot. Controlling distractions can be a factor you'll have to look out for. You may see yourself as being able to stay on task if you're alone with few distractions, but having an exuberant toddler nearby is not going to fit well in your perfect new profile life.

Even if you can secure a location within your

home that is free from outside interference, just about anyone with ADHD will fully understand that just the knowledge that someone else is nearby could be enough to pull them off point. When creating your profile these are things you need to keep in mind.

In order to create this perfect balance there are a few things that are important to keep in mind.

- Think about the time when you will do your work. If you're going to be working at home, consider scheduling your time when the kids are at school or after they go to bed. You will be in complete control of your schedule, so you don't have to stick to the 9-5 shift most have become accustomed to.
- Learn to prioritize and put things in order. If you have family responsibilities that need to be addressed, what are they? By making sure they get done first, you prepare a way for the rest of the day to go smoothly.
- Setup visual reminders. This will help you to keep things prioritized in the right order. When you have visual reminders of the most important things that need to be done in both work and family, you are less likely to get distracted and neglect some of your responsibilities.

- Create your own goals. Make sure you use S.M.A.R.T. to keep you on track. Your goals should be Specific, Measurable, Achievable, Realistic, and Time-bound.
- Curb the tendency to say yes to everything. People with ADHD will easily let their emotions and enthusiasm dictate their actions. They may agree to things impulsively and then fail to follow through later on when the excitement begins to wane. By resisting the impulse to say yes you can avoid many of the problems that will inevitably come later.
- Whenever possible, reduce distractions.
- Find a buddy to bounce ideas off of. They don't have to be in the same household or in the same neighborhood, but if you can find someone you can talk through your impulsive ideas, they can help to keep you grounded during those out of control and chaotic days. Your buddy could be a member of your family or it could be a friend on the other side of the country. Whoever you choose, regular conversations with them will help to keep you grounded.

Keep in mind, that in your goal to create your own environment, the search must extend to include your family too. This can create a whole other realm of pitfalls you'll have to take into consideration, especially if you have other people with ADHD in your household.

However, by working along with your family you can create an environment where everyone can thrive.

Of course, you will still have to be aware of your weaknesses, but once identified, you can develop strategies, plans, and situations that avoid those problems and put the majority of your focus on making your strong qualities even stronger.

When it comes to relationships, it can be very challenging if you don't have a plan. You're not just dealing with your chaotic mind but you're trying to decipher what is going on in the minds of those close to you. This becomes increasingly more difficult if your family doesn't really understand what you're going through.

Make sure that those you're close to understand that your mind craves constant stimulation and excitement. If you can find ways to help them to understand the chaos of your mind, it can go a long way in keeping the relationship from getting into trouble.

When explaining things to your family and friends, avoid using words like disorder or disability and focus on words like different and unique. The better you are able to articulate your needs the easier it will be for them to see those needs and help you to meet them.

If they are able to understand these things, they will not see your constant changes as something negative, bad, or wrong. Instead, it is just your need to become your own best friend. If you don't speak up for yourself and make your needs known, you can be pretty sure that others won't either, even those closest to you.

Communication is the key. When your friends and family understand, they are less likely to label you with negative expressions like, "he's just spacing out again," or "chill out and slow down." These may not necessarily be bad words, but they can hurt just the same. They lead to resentment and hard feelings that can take years to overcome. Your best bet is to create an environment where these things are avoided from the beginning. That way, you don't waste recovery time trying to get things back on track.

When it comes to ADHD, it is more important than ever to work with your partner. We often say harsh words with those we are closest to and with the impulsive tendencies of ADHD, it would only be a matter of time before the impulse to find a more understanding partner will take hold and your relationship could be ruined forever. By communicating from the beginning about your weaknesses and tendencies and creating a strategy that you both can work with, you can avoid many hurt feelings and painful situations that could ruin a relationship.

Find Activities That You Both Can Be Excited About

In every relationship there are always going to be activities that your partner will enjoy but you will not and vice-versa. However, if you can find activities that you both enjoy and learn how to respect your partner's right to enjoy other activities without you, it will go a long way in sealing your relationship.

Strategies to Help You Go from Off Beat to On Point

You recognize that your mind is chaotic and while you don't want to accept the labels that society has put on many people with ADHD, you can't help but recognize that the way your mind works doesn't really fit in with the cultural norms.

No matter what your belief system is where you fall on the spectrum, you need to develop coping strategies that will help you to fit in with society as a whole, otherwise you might find yourself locked out of many situations you crave to be in.

Every person with ADHD has their own unique set of strategies they use to cope with the world at large and in time, you will develop your own skills in this regard. Your means of meeting these obstacles will be developed based on your personality, circumstances, and the extent of your ADHD. The strategies listed below are designed just to get you started thinking along these lines. If you find some that work well for you and you are comfortable with, feel free to adopt them as your own, make adjustments to them, or tailor them to your unique needs. Whatever the case, you need to start building up your personal repertoire of techniques to help you to navigate the world around you.

For Disorganization:

Sometimes you have to trick yourself into getting organized. Some people will make a habit of inviting people to their home every week so that they are forced to organize and clean up to prepare for their guests. Others may choose to have a good friend come over periodically to help them to sort through everything they have accumulated over the months.

When it comes to getting tasks done, they may develop a tendency to use the out of sight out of mind strategy. To avoid this, they make sure their lives are filled with plenty of visual cues to help them remember what needs to be done in a timely fashion.

Dividing tasks into smaller sections can be very beneficial for many people. They may choose to clean their house in small stages. One day clean the living room, the next day the kitchen, and the next day the bedroom. While other people could probably get the job done in one single day, by breaking up the task in small stages, you are less likely to get overwhelmed. When your mind is ready to move on to the next task, you do so with a sense of satisfaction that you have accomplished something.

Introduce color. Whether it is a shopping list or a list of tasks that need to get done, use brightly colored paper to draw you to it. It is pretty easy to find neon post-its that can easily be put in your line of sight. You are more likely to follow up on a neon pink note than a bland white piece of paper stuck to your refrigerator.

To Control Impulsive Tendencies

Many people with ADHD will practice mindfulness to help them to curtail their tendencies to be impulsive. The more you are aware of when you are reacting to impulsiveness the better you are able to control it. Try starting each day with a session on mindfulness, focusing on your emotions and feelings when impulsive tendencies strike.

When it comes to impulsive shopping, keep a list of questions to ask yourself before you make a purchase. Do I need it? Do you really want it or do you just need to buy something? Does it really fit? Does it look good on me? It also helps to have someone with you that can verbalize these questions for you when you're shopping.

When you have an impulsive idea, try taking the time to write it down first. Save it for a few hours and if it still seems like a good idea, test it out on someone else before you decide to follow through.

To Manage Stress

Meditation can be very soothing, and music and exercise works for some people. Dancing can be a great way to ease the tension and get your hyper body to settle down.

Find a distraction that can help you to forget about the stressful situation for a little while. Listen to audio books, take a walk, watch a movie, or talk on the phone with someone.

Try to unplug. That means turn off all your technical devices and just escape for a period of time. Avoid anything that connects you to the chaos of the world.

At least you can get the idea. The list could go on and on. There is no way we could list every possible strategy but as you can see, some of these strategies are pretty easy to implement, others you may have to struggle with. In time, you'll be able to develop your own so that you can successfully redirect your mind to get back in sync with the rest of the world.

Finding Your Power in Nature

Interestingly enough, those with ADHD are not always flying on a high. Even though many of them are extremely hyper, there are times when even they will have to come back down to earth and reenergize.

Some people find that settling back and listening to soothing music can have a major calming effect. Others may turn to vegging out in front of the television and others may find taking a nice relaxing bath can do the trick. But in order to tap into your superpower, it may be necessary to take those down times to another level entirely and begin to commune with nature.

Because our lives are so incredibly on the go all
the time, we may find an amazing amount of
relief in the quiet and serenity that many
natural environments provide.

When we are out in the natural world, we feel
connected to other living beings, organic beings
that have a completely different life form. The
time spent there is a time connecting us to
where we came from and where we will one day
return.

Our bodies all have a natural rhythm that
vibrates with the unspoken surroundings of
nature. Here we are connected to an entirely
new type of world and as a result, we can give
our mind a vacation from the chaos. In nature
we can lose ourselves in the cosmos for a time
and not have to worry about the time, the job,
or anything else.

Unlike the chaos of our mind, in nature
everything is in the right place, performs at the
right time, and fades away at precisely the right
moment. It is the total opposite of chaos. We
don't see leaves growing right out of the ground
nor do we see water meandering everywhere.
Everything in nature has a place, a boundary,
and a purpose.

Taking the time to slow down and study these
inner workings activates a whole new region of
the brain so that when we return to our world,
our minds are more open, and we can see

things in an entirely new light. When we are in nature we are going back to the very basics of our existence and we get to experience "being" rather than "surviving," "struggling," or "existing."

The more time we spend in nature, we are teaching our mind to be quiet, to relax, and just stop for a minute. But to get the best results when you're in nature, you need to make a conscious effort to do more than be there. You have to take the time to really see it, to look closely at the surroundings and engage all of your senses. You'll be amazed at how rejuvenated you'll feel afterward.

Channel That Surplus Energy

For those who struggle with a hyperactivity and impulsiveness with their ADHD it could be difficult to channel that energy and redirect it in more practical ways without a clear plan of action.

It can be unnerving to find yourself confined in closed quarters when that build up of energy inside you wants to explode. It can come on suddenly and without explanation. You could be sitting quietly working on a project and then your body is suddenly filled with a surge of energy that can seem almost impossible to harness.

During the times when you're not in hyper focus you could literally feel like the Energizer Bunny and just don't know how to stop yourself. You struggle even to sit for an extended period of time at the dinner table or find yourself unable to go to sleep at night.

To handle this type of situation, one thing you need to remember is that this energy is a good thing. There is nothing wrong with that strong drive to move physically, you just need to learn a few strategies to help you channel it in the right direction.

What strategies you use will depend on the particulars of the environment. The time of day it is, the location you're in, and what needs to be done at the moment. For example, if it's 2:00 in the afternoon and you're at work, it may be a good time to take a break and burn off some of the energy in a short walk.

If you're in the middle of a project, you could channel that energy into working on the task at hand if you can get your mind in sync with your body. On the other hand, when the project is not what your mind wants to do, it may be necessary to take a more creative approach.

When you have energy and your mind is fighting to stay on task, try dividing up the work into smaller tasks with little breaks in between. Work for 15 minutes and then walk to the water cooler or go outside for a few minutes, then come back and work for another 15 minutes. Each time you do this exercise, you'll be able to extend your time on your task until you're able to keep to a regular schedule.

It is important to consider what could be triggering your energy bursts. In many cases it is stimulated by your outside environment. So, if you're surrounded by television, videos, music, or other external stimuli, try to limit your exposure. Electronics can often times be mentally stimulating so try to take some time outside without all the mechanical inputs that can consume your mind. Leave your phone at your desk and just go and commune with nature.

Find a physical component to whatever task you're doing. Even little physical activities can help to relieve some of the pent-up energy inside. If the bursts happen frequently, consider taking up an exercise or sport. Try jogging before starting your work or if you work at home, get a trampoline or a boxing bag to help you channel your inner beast.

Whenever possible, try to channel that energy into the task at hand but if not, find ways to walk away from your work and get involved in something else that will help you to expend that energy in a more positive way.

Chapter 4: Thinking Differently

All through our childhood years we're taught that in order to succeed we must conform but if you have ADHD that can be a real frightening thought. It is hard enough to maintain the slow and mundane thought processes of the rest of the world. Your mind is moving at a mile a minute while your partner's or those around you seems to be moving literally at a snail's pace. The thought of "fitting in" could leave you feeling completely overwhelmed.

It does help to understand how the brain works but that's only half the battle. Oftentimes you feel like you're literally the square peg trying to fit in the round hole. If you make yourself small enough, you may be able to squeeze yourself into the world's mold, but you'll still feel like less of the person you were meant to be, and you'll have a few bumps and bruises for your effort.

To cope with this challenge, it is important to remember that your brain works differently. When you're looking for your place in the world avoid settling for jobs that require a large amount of time dedicated to mundane tasks like reading emails, scheduling, and reading and writing. For people with ADHD, these types of tasks will take twice as long to accomplish if not more.

But understanding that ADHD minds are often more suited to creative careers, artistic flair, and problem solving you can save your self-esteem and still give you a rewarding career to show for it. Think of the people throughout history that were believed to have ADHD. DaVinci, Walt Disney, and Albert Einstein for example. Benjamin Franklin was so innovative that he created and designed thousands of new gadgets and inventions, many of them are still being used today. After years of research, it is now understood that people who tend to think in unusual and non-traditional ways are naturally more creative and problem solvers.

The reason behind it is their ability to approach a situation from a completely different angle. By seeking out careers and situations that will allow you to tap into those unique talents you can fuel your mind rather than control it. But what happens when you can't find that perfect career and you're forced to be that square peg in the round hole? Chances are you're going to have a lot of pent up frustrations and you're going to need to find a way to blow off some steam or at least ease up on the tensions.

Self-Soothing Techniques

In many cases, when a person with ADHD finds himself unable to handle frustration, disappointment, and discouragement, it can trigger a cascade of negative feelings. You may not react in the same way as everyone else, feeling sometimes oversensitive and emotional about a certain situation. When you're at work, it may become evident that you're going to have to manage your emotions yourself. Remember, because you think differently, your brain is working contrary to everyone else's so you're going to have to soothe yourself differently as well.

Not being in the right environment can easily trigger stress and tension, which can build up into pent-up energy that will need to be expended. Here are a few self-soothing techniques that can help you to manage it.

1. Avoid playing the blame game. When situations do not go as planned, it is easy to get frustrated, especially when the fault is due to your lack of attention. The more you point fingers the higher your level of stress will become. Learn to accept that it is just ADHD and move on to your next goal.

2. Get physical. Physical activity is more than just getting your body moving. It also increases the level of serotonin in the brain, which is a natural stress reliever. Research shows that 30 minutes of exercise can keep you relaxed for at least a couple of hours. Taking a walk in the neighborhood, around your building, or getting moving can ease a lot of your stress.

3. Monitor your time. Quiet things rarely get the attention of someone with ADHD. Get a watch or set a timer on your computer to ring at specific intervals (every 30 minutes or every hour). It will help you to stay on task. If your alarm is your signal that you can shift to something else, you can build up the discipline to stay on task a little longer when you know that you won't need to remain there indefinitely.

4. Tap into your senses. Whether it's the power of smell, a change of scenery, playing soothing sounds, or the sensation of touch, using your senses to soothe your mind is an age-old practice that has been beneficial for all cultures, especially for those with ADHD. Aromatherapy, closing your eyes and listening to soft music, or practicing

yoga can do wonders for the mind and
the spirit.

Whenever you try any of these self-soothing
techniques, you'll have to learn how to block
out everything around you, at least for a few
minutes. Be mindful of everything around you
but don't give into them. You don't need to
spend a great deal of time doing these things. A
few minutes here, a little time there, and you'll
feel like a whole new person.

In time, you'll come up with your own
strategies to calm your anxiety. This is so
important for those with ADHD as it can really
help you to tap into your inner gifts that are
often overlooked when trying to fit into an
uncomfortable environment.

Dare to Use Your Emotions

Most people think of impulsivity and
hyperactivity when they think of ADHD but
there is another very important element that
may often be overlooked: emotions. It is very
common to suffer from runaway emotions that
when unchecked can damage relationships,
steal your thunder, and lead to making rash
decisions. Learning how to manage them can
be a very valuable resource you will be able to
rely on a great deal.

There are two sides to the emotions of ADHD. When those with ADHD are upset and angry it can be very extreme, but they will put an equal amount of energy into being very happy and excited. Either way, it can lead to negative consequences, so it is important to be able to tone down the intensity of your emotions in order to be more effective in your day-to-day activities.

There are three basic principles behind emotional self-control.

- Manage stress
- Develop strategies to control your emotions or manage the situations that may become emotional triggers
- Own your emotions

By setting these three principles as your goal, you can make a mental note to keep a watchful eye out when emotions begin to get out of control.

We already talked about managing stress earlier but here are just a few more tips that can help you to regain emotional control.

1. Try to avoid overextending yourself. This leads to time stress and the fear of disappointing those who rely on you.
2. Get enough rest.

3. Get regular exercise.
4. Avoid situations that may trigger your emotions.
5. Have a buddy or partner to talk you down when you get out of control.
6. Try to get the other person's perspective.
7. Mentally separate your feelings from your actions.

These strategies seem to be very simple but believe me, when you're in the heat of an emotional outburst they can prove to be a difficult challenge to overcome. By practicing these things on a daily basis, even with very small things, you'll be emotionally strong enough to handle the big things when they come through.

Principles to Live By

At the heart of every ADHD strategy there are some basic principles to live by. Rules only work in very specific situations but by understanding a universal truth that will help you to tailor your strategies to your unique set of circumstances they can serve as a guiding light helping you to find that perfect environment conducive to your ADHD. Follow these principles and you're good to go.

1. Make sure boundaries are visible outside of your mind so you can see them,

stimulating more of your senses in your decision-making process.
2. When consequences result from an impulsive action, address it immediately.
3. Switch up your reward system so your mind does not tire of the same thing.
4. Anticipate problems and be proactive in addressing them. In situations where the same problem keeps coming up, create a plan to address it before it arises again.
5. Channel your energy in positive directions.
6. Tap into your creativity and seek out situations where you can use your ADHD in positive ways.

Chapter 5: Managing Your Time With ADHD

Because of the chaotic state of the mind and the impulsive nature, adults with ADHD often struggle with managing time well. Their natural tendency to be restless and impulsive makes it difficult to concentrate on anything for an extended period of time. As a result, they may not be aware of the passing of time, may not be able to gauge exactly how long a task will take, and have an inability to adjust their activities to stay within a particular time frame.

For that reason, it is important for them to learn a few time management strategies that will help them to overcome this weakness and get tasks done in a timely manner. Some of the strategies listed here are basic and can apply in almost any situation but there are others that may be a little more unique. Pick and choose those that will work best for you and adjust them to your personal circumstances.

Time Management in Everyday Situations

- To-Do Lists: To-do lists are more than just about maintaining a daily reminder of what needs to be done. It is also a means of visual stimulation. The lists simply access another one of your senses, which helps to reinforce your ability to stay on task. The trick to making this work is to keep the list small, only including the most important tasks on it. Too long of a list and you'll find yourself being overstimulated, which would work contrary to your goals.

- Use color-coding in your notes: For the person with ADHD, setting priorities that you can stick to can be very difficult. Keeping in line with tapping into other senses to keep you on time can be very beneficial. By listing the things you need to do by color, you can easily prioritize the more important things in a more prominent color and the less important tasks can be in more subtle colors. Others may choose to code their tasks by the time of day they need to be done. Things that must be completed in the morning may be in red, afternoon yellow, and the evening could be coded in blue. Create your own color-coding system and make sure it is someplace where it can catch your eye frequently.
- Don't overschedule. Make sure that you have set aside a realistic amount of time to accomplish what you set out to do. Factor in how much time it may take you to get started on a task in order to determine if it is feasible enough to even

attempt. Procrastination is a big part of ADHD life, so you need to think about the time you won't be working on it, too. Your goal is to avoid the mad frenzy of activity you may have as you near the finish line.

- Set alarms: Audio reminders on your computer, your watch, smart phone, tablet, or any other device can help to reel you back in when you've drifted off track. ADHD people do not have a reliable internal clock, so you will need to create an external one you can depend on.

In your enthusiasm, you may find that you often bite off more than you can chew. To prevent that from happening, create a schedule that includes plenty of small break times so that you don't get bored. When that happens, your instances of distractions can be strong. When the work is done in small bite sized pieces you eliminate the possibility of the mind needing to switch gears to re-stimulate itself.

Set Time Management Goals

Those with ADHD often have only two ways to view time. For them it is either running too fast, they are in a desperate scramble to catch up or it's running too slow and they struggle to keep their minds on task. This can be a tough obstacle to overcome but by setting a few time management goals, you can "trick" your brain into keeping better time.

These goals will give you a strong sense of purpose that will fortify your spirit. It's not enough to know that you need to be on time, finish work on time, or pick up the kids on time; the most powerful motivator of all is when you know why so gear your time management goals with that in mind and you'll automatically become more time conscious. Here are a few tips you can use to tap into your inner resources and help you stay on time.

1. **It's Empowering:** When you can manage your time better you find you are in control. This gives you the power to dictate how you spend your day, which will naturally help you to alleviate stress, boost your self-esteem, and calm that inner beast.
2. **It's More Efficient:** When you're in control you are more likely to be more efficient. You will be more productive and will be able to accomplish more.
3. **It Puts Your Goals Within Reach:** Time management is an effective motivator. As you are able to accomplish more, your goals will be more achievable. Nothing can be more stimulating than when you see a long-term goal getting closer and closer by

the day simply because you have managed your time better.

4. **It Gives You a Sense of Satisfaction:** When you manage your time, you have to strike a balance between what's important and what's not. While your mind will want to drift from the more important tasks to those that are more fun and engaging, that sense of fulfillment is what will bring you back in line. Success in this area will be rewarding and a strong motivator for you to stick to those things that are more important. The feeling is like a drug and you'll definitely want to experience more of it.

Time management is probably one of the most important skills you can develop to help manage your ADHD. It will give you a sense of balance and teach you how to spend your time and spread out your energy so that you don't over stimulate or burn out from the chaos that's running your mind. In short, it will give you a more stable and consistent quality of life that will take you a long way.

Chapter 6: Taking it to the Next Level

In the beginning of this book, we talked about creating an environment that would be better suited for someone with ADHD. We discussed different types of jobs that someone with a chaotic mind may be more drawn to and have a higher potential for success.

Those are the ideal situations where you have an employer and co-workers who are willing to adjust their work lives and schedules to meet your needs. These situations can be a true lifesaver for someone with ADHD, but they are not always easy to come by. Some people with ADHD may not be able to fit well into any work environment and may feel frustrated no matter what type of accommodations are made for them.

It is a natural tendency for someone with ADHD to want to strike out on their own. In fact, according to some reports, adults with ADHD are 300% more likely to want to leave the constraints of a traditional working environment behind and strike out on their own.

It is the one avenue that seems to pull at the heartstrings of many. It serves their creative juices, their desire to create a world that is molded by their minds, and it gives them the freedom to not have to conform to a society that goes contrary to their nature.

If you're thinking along these lines, you're in good company. Many people have thought the same exact thing and have made the attempt. Unfortunately, many have also failed at the prospect; their impulsive nature caused them to jump first, and then try to swim for the surface.

They fell into a common trap. While most people with ADHD are better suited for entrepreneurship, it is rare that they will succeed without factoring in some crucial details.

Allow for Distractions

The ADHD mind will always be distracted no matter what kind of work you do. Create a business that will be flexible enough for you to step out from time to time and change directions.

Many set up new business situations that literally trap them in an endless cycle from which they cannot extricate themselves. When your business demands your time 24/7, you do not allow for your natural tendency to crave a change of scenery.

Of course, in the beginning you'll need to dedicate more time and money to get started but make sure your goals and directions are focused on keeping you flexible, so you can remove yourself when you need to.

Give the Business a Direction

You need a specialty that taps into your creative talents. When you start, make sure it is focused to serve a specific public and meet a unique need that only your talents can provide. As the business becomes more successful, you can expand if you wish. So, whether you're planning on a catering business or designing a new app for smart phones, keep the business going steadily forward in a single direction.

You Can Wear Several Hats, but Don't

Any new business requires the owner/manager to wear several hats and your ADHD tendency will encourage you to do that. But this may lead to you getting overwhelmed with too much work to do and you end up stalling out like a flooded engine in your car.

Allow for help to come in and take on the more mundane tasks of running a business so your mind is free to continue to create and produce.

When you hire people, be clear when giving them directions. Give them detailed job descriptions and make sure that you communicate to them exactly what is expected. Include a list of skills needed for each job and make sure that you hire the right people for the job you require.

Use Your Visual Cues

The same visual cues you needed to home in your mental faculties when you were learning to manage your ADHD are the same ones you'll need to manage a business, just bigger. You'll be in charge of not just your own actions but of those who work for you.

When creating these cues, make sure that you keep it simple enough for anyone to follow it. Set standards and stick to them. When you can do all of these things, the beauty of running a business that allows you to be free cannot be within reach.

What Kind of Business to Start?

Now that you have an idea of how to get started, you need to think about the type of business you want to start. It's not as easy as you might think. With minds that are all over the place, have an impulse to move, and a drive to be in complete control, there are a lot of moving parts that need to be considered.

To choose the right business for you, you will have to learn how to think outside of the box. You need to understand the inner regions of your mind, your unique skills and talents, and the society you want to insert them in.

First, think of a problem in the community that needs to be solved and then determine if you have the creativity, talent, and skills to offer a solution. Your advantage here is that your unique mind doesn't problem solve like other minds. Your strengths will be more inclined in finding completely new ways to approach an old problem. You have actually been pre-programmed to look at situations differently and as a result you'll tap into an area that the rest of the world has yet to discover.

Use that idea to create a business that will service that public need and set about starting your own plan. Choose those things that you know give you satisfaction and you have had fun doing. By tapping into the unique mind you have been given and harnessing that mind in positive ways, you can launch your life into a whole new stratosphere and literally end up using your ADHD as your personal superpower that will launch you into a whole new and profitable career you can really be proud of.

Conclusion

Thanks for making it through to the end of this book, let's hope it was informative and able to provide you with all of the tools you need to achieve your goals whatever they may be.

When you have ADHD, you crave stimulus from your environment. That stimulus could come in the form of family, work, or social events or it could come from nature itself. Unlike the days of the past where survival depended largely on whether or not you could conform to a predetermined mode of behavior in society.

Fast forward today, those with ADHD have a wealth of opportunities to take advantage of. These are the kind of people that will find more satisfaction from a hard day's work that taps into their best gifts and talents rather than shuffled behind a desk or performing mundane tasks.

You don't need to get rid of your energy to be successful, you simply need to channel it in the right direction to create your own personal environment. And if you can't find the right spot for you in this world, create your own. Now, what kind of world is that to live in?

We live at a very opportune time, a time when we can choose our lives a la carte and the perfect lifestyle for the one who chooses to take advantage of it, and the ideal answer to many of the challenges that those with ADHD face daily. Armed with the right tools, anything is possible.

Finally, if you found this book useful in anyway, a review on Amazon is always appreciated!

www.ingramcontent.com/pod-product-compliance
Lightning Source LLC
Chambersburg PA
CBHW051227250726
48655CB00006B/2636